HIDDEN, RACISM AND THE GLBT MOVEMENT

ANEB JAH RASTA SENSAS-UTCHA NEFER I

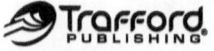 www.trafford.com
North America & international
toll-free: 1 888 232 4444 (USA & Canada)
fax: 812 355 4082

Within this particular movement there are several important health and spiritual factors that must be recognized, comprehended as well as dealt with. First of all; in Autoandrophilia, in which an assigned female at birth is sexuall aroused by the thought of being a man, behaving as a man while playing the role of a man while involved in a lesbian relationship. You see, the ancient Greeks who considered the Egyptians and Canaanites great, yet considered the paganistic outwardly, consider the following; (self) - (man) fear of one's self as a man is called AutoAndrophobia. This is where estrogen levels have been contraindicated due to deep vein thrombosis and antiandrogens.

This is an estrogen and testosterone inbalance due to medical and spiritual self harm of the Schizotypal behavior. This type of individual has caused harm to itself through superstition worshipping. This is an allegorical form of worshipping by the the scheming schemers. Also, note; In the aspects of Herukhuti and Heru according to the Khamitic Tree of Life the two are male. However; the female worships the two in order of fulfilling their own perverted lusts. This is where gay domination, lesbianism and gayism occurs and the two terms that are listed above Autoandrophilia and Autoandrophobia take place. Whereas; they consider themselves as muscle gods.

Therefore; you will see that this book will cover everything from a brief history of hidden messages that have been written in western education, health, religion and spirituality. In addition; psychiatry of Christianity, Judaism and Islam.

Also, in addition hypothalamic disorders cause several forms of Pituitary tumors and aneurysms due to other medical conditions. Therefore; within the GLBT there is a chronic disturbance of their brain cells. The brain cells become traumatized due to an inconsistent and hypocratical religious and spiritual system. There's no magic button towards one being healed for mental illnesses and other diseases. If you have no understanding of a belief system don't claim it.

Seek counsel! Deuteronomy 28:28 The Lord will inflict with madness, blindness and confusion of the mind. Therefore: many people are limited in their thinking to surface and external experiences that they cannot determine differences of biological, physiological or spiritual support for GLBT sex. Metu Neter Volume 1 page 104 mentions exactly what was stolen by the Romans in the 1st Chapter of Romans verse 24 - 27!

First of all; Individuals who cannot determine physiological and or biological differences between sexes do so on their own behalf. This is mere madness and confusion of the mind as written in the book of Deuteronomy 28:28. You see; madness is through insane forms of delusion as well as psychiatrical fantasies. Within these fantasies individuals tend to ruin and or speed up patterns of their brain by compulsions towards daydreaming and focusing on the externalizied factors of irrational thinking.

There is no biological, physiological and or spiritual support for the GLBT. Also; one must take into account that there is no religious context that permits this form of immorality. However; there is spiritual suppor for the confused, mentally blind and madness of individual with psychiatric disorders. However; it is westernized. westernized in every form of mythology. In mythology, its scholars have excluded the facts that Egyptologists have gotten it so wrong in their quest to undermind the people of The Promise Lands {the seven nations of Canaan} with derogatory forms of intellectualism with regards to the greatness.

Written in the Kaballah by A.E. Waite on page 329 the following; "it is added that those who know this sexual mystery will be in position to see why the Holy Land was given a patrimony to Canaan before the coming of the Hebrew Israelites". They have painted and tainted pictures regarding the nations of Canaan, Kemet and all of Africa as being monkies and of sexual prowess. They've also mentioned tha Blacks are illerate, meader, ignorant, violent and are a paganistic race of people.

Their colonizing tactics and words have worked considerably. Whereas; words have power. They can germinate a people towards a greater form of anxiety, delusion, depression, self-denial, self-hatred, crime and suicide. This includes taking part within the GLBT Movement! For; they are incarcerated within the GLBT Movement!

HIDDEN RACISM'S WITH ETERNAL LIES

The purpose of African history is to promote group self-esteem towards the African people. This is due to the fact that the African heritage has been hidden from the African people. In most cases, by the clergy / Black Clergy. In many cases, those who lack knowledge of the origins will fall for anything that other races and cultures present to them. By all means, this is an example of the fool being enslaved by the slaver. Mary Lefkowitz and other so-called Egyptologists, historians and scholars of African culture, / race relations have their heads in the dark clouds of darkness. She's a bigot and a racist. Whereas; in her book "Not Out of Africa", she's in constant denial of her racist ambitions.

That is to fool her constituents "Caucasians and blind African Americans that she's not a bigot and or blind illacious woman.

Lefkowitz has not studied the philosophers of Greece nor African ancestry. Neither has she studied African historians of the past and present. Therefore; her knowledge and understanding is delusional. It is unfair to mention that the African Race received its knowledge from Greece, Rome and Europe. However, it is the opposite. The Bible was written for the Catholic, Greek, Jew and Christian slaver in order to manipulate the lower- being of the meek.

They have no knowledge of the origin of their religion. They have no evidence of it. Neither do they have knowledge of the origin of what they are to have faith in. The Aunkh cross is an electromagnetic device that represents the balancing and the unifying of the creation of life. That is, man and woman. In this, CPR and the AED - Automation External Defibulator machine is used to assist in the healing of individuals who have a loss of consciousness. This is to provide energy through current and shock. In such as the Aurisa Aunk of the Paut Neteru. This is within the Kamitic Tree of Life. Also, note that this is somewhat similar to the Yin and the Yin of the Chinese zodiac and calander

The defibulator will say "shock". Shock is a word of power. Whereas; individuals will be faced with the head - tilt- chin - lift syndrome. Check for consciousness, a pulse and breathing. You see, the African Race has been demoralized by the Rosy Cross and its lop-sided questioning with regards to its testing procedures and left-brained testing requirements. This is similar the The Mental Measurements that have been created by The Buros Institute which is located in Nebraska.

What are the following; cerebral palsy, TB, Lupus, Hepititis, diabetes, epilepsy and seizures? They all can be determined by shock with regards to sudden forms of excitment which leads to sudden trauma. The skin turns pale, moist and or grayish. There is also restlessness, lack of consciousness, rapid breathing and or excessive thirst. In this, while providing CPR to an infant, child or adult -, there are a variety of different steps and procedures that must occur. There is a difference between a one and two rescuer as well as a conscious and unconscious individual.

1 rescuer of an unconscious person / child / adult requires 30 chest compressions and 2 rescue breaths - perform cpr. 1 rescuer of a conscious person requires you to perform 30 chest compressions along with 2 chest compressions. Note: techniques for adult - child choking. Whereas; the conscious and unconscious infant - 1 and 2 rescuer differs in procedural techniques. 15 chest compressions and two rescue breaths for an infant. 5 back blows and 5 chest compressions for choking individuals. includes choking and non-choking, conscious / unconscious infant. Check the brachial artery. Give chess compressions two minutes prior to using the AED.

Compression depth 3 inches Adult, 2 inch child 1 1/2 inch for infant

Also, within certain communities, and environments where there's poverty and uncertainty. In urban areas this is very seldom taught. Whereas; individuals lack knowledge, uninformed or are just dependent on EMS to provide services for those who are in special need of care.

The Egyptologists, Arabs, Europeans, Jews and Christians have epistilized ancient Kemet by shaming it with doctrines of intellectualisms of the Setien. This is to say, with its hidden forms of racism and discrimination by dehumanizing minorties throughout the world. The Setien is the world system of mercantilism and slavery of every kind! By the way, where are the tombs of Mohammed and Jesus? We know that the Egyptians built the pyramids and they had tombs. They are an envied people. Therefore; lies are eternal. Islam and Christianity are eternal lies that are filled with delusion and psychotic forms of granduer. This leads to maniacal forms of uncivilized behavioral patterns. It is obvious that this is organized racism.

This form of racism has been also initialized from the caucasian unto the African - African American. In this, there has been a great deal of brainwashing at the hands of the holier-than-nowers of Christianiaty and Islam. They memorize scripture. However, they deny the healing powers of God / Self - within. This is, they deny the manifestations of God that are within them. They seek external means of the divine. They are hippocrates, thieves, GLBTs, con artists and liars. Western religion has pit the black male against the black woman and vise/versa. The Holy Bible is contrary within itself.

An Afrocentric Guide To A Spiritual Union by Ra Un Nefer Amen I / Public Enemy: Revolutionary Generation 1990

You see, the true origins and history of the African civilization has never fully been told and recognized by the clergy, healthcare, psychiatry and educational systems since their origin. In this, mental illness and learning disabilities often occur. The United States Dept. of Education is negligent as a result of its irregular forms and methods regarding its rules and regulations according to race relations. This includes the lack of civil rights, racial equality and the hidden forms of discriminatory practices within the levels of preschool to post-secondary training. Those manic behaviors will eventually and has triggered within the mindset of teenagers, future adults as well as teachers, professors and individuals within all areas of professions.

It is said, "faith is the substance of things hoped for, but are unseen. Whereas; There are over 14,800 versions of the Bible that are only words of men. Every man is a liar. Indeed, this is Romanticisms by the Euro-Greco-Roman as it is written in Romans 1:20. Invisible things are clearly seen, being understood by the things that are made, even his eternal power and eternal Godhead. This is eternal damnation as many know what they want. They are are in pursuit therof. Therefore; the people are without excuse. In this, homosexuality is an eternal sin against the eternal nature of God that leads to eternal damnation. The entire first chapter of Romans issues messages regarding homosexality and idol worship. Those acts are committed secretly. Behind closed doors of the wicked and evil witches and devils of illusion. Deliberate sin is unforgivable.

Also, It says in Numbers 23:9, I see a people who do not even know themselves. Therefore; we, the African civilization and children have been blinded and blindsided by hidden forms of shame, doubt, hatred, discrimination and racism. You see, a nation is a large aggregate of people united by common decent, history, culture and or language; inhabiting in a particular country or territory. This includes nations that promote GLBTQ communities, sexism and racisms.

However the history of Africa has been stolen by European and Arab invasions along with whoremongers of idolatry. These are trangressions that are and have been hidden and uncurable due to a constant disobedience of the forceful and arrogant factors of the disobedience.

Therefore; Proverbs 14:34 Righteousness exalts a nation but sin condemns any people. In addition, all have mental and spiritual conditions that can trigger amongst others within the same nation, community and spiritual klan / nation. Individuals have been known to commit intentional sin in order to please and sooth their own spiritual, behavioral and mental conditions. This is wickedness and hatred towards the Creator of the universe.

You see, this is where imitation occurs. Individuals learn from conditioned patterens of subliminal messages. These messages can be intentional and or uninvited. However, in most cases, they are pathogens of delusion and scheme. This is invoked within an induviduals being and eventually decreases ones ability to maintain a higher and stable living pattern. Your lower being is then invoked by those of whom you have confided with.

In addition, everyone, people are distinct with their own right. They have the right to choose their lifestyle.

However; God ignors the foolish, wise arrogant and hippocrate as a result of their intentional wrondoings. They are only fooling themselves by their cleverness of wickedness. They are attempting to fool you. Beware of them! I must say! They are haters of God and lovers of idolatry. I will continue this party of convicting the GLBTQ and racist bigot of whom I am imprisoned by. For, they take kindness for weakness. Their intentions are to kill steal and destroy ones righteousness.

Whereas; everyone is his or her own nation. A nation of sublime and unique culture within itself. Therefore; seek counsel! For you have no understanding of yourselves. You cannot become weak in order to make someone else strong. Therefore; I am not a Christian, Muslim or Jew. However; they say the following and refuse to live up to their own doctrines. Isaiah 59:2 Your sins have seperated you from the creator. Your sins have hidden his face from you, so that he will not hear.

Luke 8:17 All things that are hidden will be revealed in light. Therefore; the foolish things are used to confound by the wise. Surah 7: 80-81 Lot said to his people: Do you commit an abomination which no one in the world did before you? Surely, you come to males with lust instead of females. Nay, you are a people of exceeding bounds. 26: 165-166 Do you come to males from amongst the creatures and leave your wives whom your lord created for you. Lot too was an incesting being of Sodom who had sexual intercourse with his two daughters. The two daughters bore sons who were later to be known as the Moabites and Ammonites.

However, in the New Testament of the Bible 2 Peter 2: 7-8 it says that the lord delivered Lot and considered him a holy man. This is contrary towards the history of the African people and civilization. Judaism and Christianity has devoured the souls of the African civilization with its loquatious excuses and hippocratical messages / hearsays regarding individuals being forgiven and saved. Indeed, why wasn't Canaan pardoned as Moses was granted the right to conquer the above people and nations for reasons of hatred along with the pride of Judaism that is documented in Exodus 3 and Genesis Chapter 9. Whereas; Moses, Miriam and Aaron were born in Egypt, North Africa during the reign of Meri-Ra Pepi I during the 6th Dynasty.

{Read later regarding the Promise Land}

Throughout the countries of the continent of Africa the GLBT movement is considered and abomination. An abomination is a serious violation or offense against God. Also, individuals have been murdered, slaughtered, tortured and or maimed for those vile acts.

Therefore: Racism, religion, neurology and psychiatry are no mysteries unto humankind. However, they are. The African race has always been depicted as animals and heathens by the Christian, Jew, Greek, Arab, Caucasian and Egyptologist. Yes, they have hidden the truth with regards to the greatness of the / our African heritage by Europeanizing, Arabizing and Christianizing the ancestry of our people. Therefore, whenever the truth is spoken about African culture, heritage, race and origins it is considered an opinion. However; whenever someone denounces Africa as a nation of heathens and pagans it is considered fact. That is to say; the African nations and people have been deceived by the establishment of the fraudulent systems of the ponzy scheming educational assessments of the western civilization.

The Bible is the top selling book. However, The Holy Bible was written by a criminalizing people. Those people were delusional and they had a God complex! There's no factual evidence of its characters - (people). There are no archeological facts of its characters, their history or heritage. It is a book of themes and stories of fables, folktales and inconsistencies regarding culture, race, laws and themes. You see, decentralization is not only modern. It occurred during the times and writings of Judaism, Christianity and Islam. It is a known fact that you have deceived the Black while continuing to come into contact. This might seem like a tape recorder within my writings. Hovever, it is a known fact regarding the revelation of wickedness and the demoralizing of our ancestry by the non-African. You are not understanding of getting my message.

Truly, they've psychologically observed us, studied us and trained us into their conditions of socialization and decivilization by the institutionalization of slavery and servitude. Portugal, / Spain and the Berber who were the Moors of Morocco, enslaved western Africans by introducing and inducing them with the hatred of the modernized methods of Catholicism, Christianity - Judaism and Islam. Their teachings were of the Roman writer, Tertullian and Constantine, the ruler of the Byzantine Empire. This is the promotion homosexuality and lewdness.

You see, they invoke you into their realm of emotion, thought and compatability by deharmonizing your lower being. Meaning, you are being monitored so they they could make you a form of their operant conditioning. They steal your being by eating your lower being. Whereas; Ephesians 6:5 aids the promotion of slavery. Slaves obey your earthly masters with respect and fear, and with sincerity of the heart, just as you would obey Christ!

Galatians 6:13 they glory off of your flesh so that you can be circumcised in order to save them. Moreover, the biblical writers and Egyptologists knew better. For they have gone on to maniplate the lowly, due to racism and discrimination. This is due to their prudence and arrogance towards those who were and are considered to be limited in the following areas; wisdom, knowledge, understanding and education. This is due to them, the lowly facing chastisement during and after the movement of enslavement and spiritual captivity.

Ephesus is in Greece. Whereas; Apostle Paul knew better. For, he was once King Saul in the Old Testament. Therefore; on February 8, 1857 - / a sermon by former president of the LDS, Brigham Young. This article was printed on February 18, 1857 by Deseret News is as follows; He cannot attain to it without the shedding of his blood. Blood Atonement! Is there a man or woman who would say, "shed my blood that I might be exalted with the Gods". This is similar the Alqaeda, Boko Haram, Isis and The Islamic Jihad.

Therefore, which gods was he speaking of? This is contrary to it's own teeth. You see, in various parts of the Old Testament this thing is forbidden. See Deuteronomy 12:31. In addition, Apostle Paul confirms that he was a master of Judaism in Galatians NIV - 1:19 I was advancing in Judiasm beyond many of my own age among my people and was extremely zealous for the traditions of my fathers. Saul too was a murderer. So you tell me you want forgiveness regarding the actions taken against the African Race and other innocent people and nations.

Therefore; the meek and humble are used as sacrifices and for catering the sensual neeeds and passions of others while they -/ themselves suffer unwanted miseries of hostilities, pain, discrimination, poverty and other forms of suffering.

In addition; the LDS (restoration) had gotten it's origin from the Egyptians of ancient Khamit. In this, they deny the manifestations of Ausar. Whereas; man is created in the image and likeness of God. However, in ancient Egypt there were no forms of sacrificial atonement upon others within that particular land until the entering of Gnostisim, the Arab, Christian and Jewish religions. They had come into contact with them by invasion and settlement. As they were all of gayisms, hatred and murderous in nature.

You see, hidden means that something is being out of sight, concealed, unseen and invisible. In this, there can be hidden forms of disease, mental illness, drug addiction, perverse addictions, homosexuality, racism and hatred. This is within the neurological realm and scope of the entire brain. Especially, its minor portions that are often unrecognized as to having disorders and dysfunctions.

Ireneaus of Gaul now, Rome used the teachings of Apostle Paul in his messages. However, the people of Gaul were cannibals. As Critognatus was a Celt in the fulfilling of Ceasar's quest of endocannibalism. In this, Transmissible Spongiform Encepholapathy TSE's are prion diseases that affects the brain and nervous system of animals and humans. 5th BCE, Hippocrates described a disease like TSE in cattle and sheep.

Prion diseases are pathogens that are within our current areas of neuroscience, health and medicine. You see, Fatal Familial Insomnia FFI is a rare autosomal dominant inherited prion disease that is caused by mutation of protein. In this, there is also disorders of the mammillian portion of the brain. Animal behaviors occur within those who monitor the dreams of others. Yet they observe ones dreams and later obstruct their present and future. Whereas; they are seteins who are seeking whom they can devour. 1 Peter 5:8 Satan seeks whom he may devour.

In most cases, there's no insomnia. There are deceitful individuals with the evil intentions of obstruction, disaster and destruction towards the sensitive and caring individuals of the world. They've aroused their animal behaviors to the point of murdering individuals while they are still alive. As death is dying to someone or some hidden life-forces that are invoked by khaibet forms of passion by the depressed, lonely, GLBTQ community and the sahu spirited personality. This goes along with hidden agendas of segregation and racism.

Medications also invoke triggers as well as maniacal behaviors and conditions that distrupt an individuals opportunity for and towards the successes that are within their realm. You see, there are brains within the brain that are invoked by patterns of stimuli. This stimuli can be evaluated by the segregative portion of the brain. In addition, the mammallian brain causes manic episodes and a variety of delusional forms of graduer. The Phi Complex of the brain allows the coordination of behavior to be evaluated.

Also, in aggression, this causes hatred towards the oppsite sex, sexual aggression and sexual addiction that leads to and is a result of idleness, low self-esteem, substance abuse, jealously, homophobia, hatred, racism and crime. Substance and medication abuse causes disorientation of gender. This is also due to an individual being narcissistic and histrionicly delusioned by his or her own actions and motives. They are also induced with PTSD. This is when they become scapegoats by blaming their negative behavioral traits and sins on others.

The Aaronic / Moses Syndrome has become a dialog to promote false religions and hippocratical religious, spiritual and political leaders for thousands of years. Therefore; Prion diseases are a result of hatred, arrogance and racisms.

In addition, animal diets tend to cause neurological diseases. Morturary Cannibalism causes Kuru as children and the elderly were fed portions of the human brain. This began in Northern Europe, Great Britian, Germany and in the nation of Gaul. This tradition was passed on unto the Fore Tribe of Papua, New Guinea as European scholars have failed to mentioned. This was written in my previous book. "Racism With Substance Induced Mood Disorders".

In this, Transmissible Spongiform Encephalopathy occurs. This causes various difficulties in speech and stool elimination. This also causes tremors with unsteady stance and gait. Therefore, there have been infections within the entire nervous system which includes both the Pineal and Pituitary Glands. This is when Parkinson's and diseases of the liver occurs. This is caused by Alcoholism, the use of anti-psychotic, anti-anxiety medications as well as antidepressants!

Hormone melatonin disorders within the pineal gland include sexual dysfunction, peptic disorders and major depressive disorder. In addition, the locus coerules that is within the brainstem is involved with the physiological responses to anxieties, panic disorders and PTSD.

Therefore, in experimental medicine of the embryonic development of (BBB) Blood-Brain Barrier during animal toxicology there have been forms of retardation in rabbits. Onauniform diet has been advised for animals and individuals within the Sickel Anemia. African Americans received Onauniform as treatment.

Animal toxicology, in most cases are similar to experimental healthcare and medicine. This includes racism, sexism, genderism and the GLTB,,,,,,,,,,

PARAPSYCHOLOGY & FOREKNOWLEDGE

F oreknowledge and parapsychology are somewhat similar. The two words are to inform us that things can be revealed through prophecy, wisdom and or through psychic abilities. Therefore; how does a particular disorder or disease occur? Whereas; they say that Robert Gallo - created activity in the guide to the HIV / Aids Virus research in 1984. Also note that this is a travesty resulting from human error that other STD's have occurred. Whereas; in chemical and biological warfare agents that were and are still being used towards, minorities, Africans, Hatians and individuals in the military -/ This has been a conspiracy to commit genocide against a particular people, the meek. However;

the GLBT agenda and drug abuse nation / culture has demoralized themselves by committing vile acts of idolatry and methods of inappropriate conditioning.

Gender Europoria and issues of transvalism has deluted the kingdom of creation prior to the enslavement of The African. The European was and still is a wild ravenous pig. In this, there is a form of disporia in the mainstream of western philosophy and culture. Many have fallen for this form of racial inequality that has triggered various diseases upward and onward by the lies of the mainstream of wickedness and evil. The intent to enslave mentally the blind and unschooled within the mainstrean of westernized forms of institutionalized education.

The House-Negroe, Caucasian and western religions such as Islam, Catholicism, Christianity and Judaism are filled with lusts, perversions as well as extreme forms of psychotic emotions that aren't written in the Diagnostic Statistical Manual (DSM). Those energies are electrofied with a variety of systems of delusion and grandios methods of GLBTQ traditions of men, women, boys and girls. Deuteronomy 16:19 For they have perverted justice with their perverted passions and false forms of compassion. They have caused mankind to self-destruct. That is to say, "commit genocide by fooling itself"

The mystery-making and demonizing effect of White Supremacy has incarcerated the mind of the African Geneology by making women into men and men into punks / faggots. Within the Hadith it is written that "if a woman comes upon another woman - the both of them are adulteresses. When a man mounts upon another man, the throne of god shakes. Kill the one that is doing it and kill the one that is is being done to. You see, this has been in existence since the European, Jew and Arab has come into contact with the African civilization. This includes the writing of the Holy Bible and Quran. They have been used in order to form a war angainst the indigenous people wherever they are natives.

James 2:9 Beware of personal favortism. If you show favortism, you sin and are convicted by the law as transgressors of the universal laws that governs all living organisms. In this, they know what they do. However; Luke 23:34 Jesus said "Father forgive them; For they know not what they do"! Were they forgiven? Are they forgiven! Have you fallen in the same categorical form of reprisal. Fallen from grace with your use of the WICCA and soothsaying personalities in order to scheme upon the lower being of individuals with a continued mass of false justifications. These justifications are to only satisfy yourselves with carnal delusionals that are filled with passions of adultry, homophobia, lies, merchandise, scheme, hatred, suicide and murder.

Therefore; Ezekiel 18:4 All souls are mine. The soul of the father is mine so is the soul of the son. The soul that sinneth shall see death. Surah 17: 75-77 as well as the male aspects of Seker with regards to the Kemetic Tree of Life,,,, St. John mentioned in Revelations 20:10 that the dead were judged according to their works. This was derived from ancient Khamit's third sphere of the Tree of Life. The male aspects of Seker judges the dead who have lived in a disharmonizing lifestyle that had been contrary to the divine and universal laws and God. Therefore, are you really going to heaven. Whereas; your behaviours, attitudes, emotions and conditions determine whether or not you are on heaven while you are living on earth as well as your destination afterlife.

In the Bible of the Jew and Christian, Matthew 6:33 it says, But seek first the kingdom of God and His rightcheousness and all things will be given unto you.

Job 2:9 Job's wife told him to hold on to his integrity and also told him to curse God and die. Therefore, they are scoffers. They invoke God in order to steal from God and eventually and constantly obstruct God from pursuing his own personal visions. They attempt to invoke obstructive, psychological and physiological conditions and behavior patterns of maniacal treasons upon HIM with conspiring and seductive spirits.

Earlier in the Book of Job, Job 2:7 says that Satan went out from the presence of the Lord. Therefore; there are setiens that attempt to equate the LGBT with the Black struggle. This cannot be done. Whereas; the Black struggle is for human and civil rights. On the otherhand; the GLBT movement is a struggle to enhance their ability to continue their inhumane behaviors. This is when the Western civilization tends to prostitute itself for any form of gain. Whether it is through employment, econimical, fair housing and or political.

In addition, The Mary Lefkowitz Sybdrome has poisoned humanity. If you have an understanding of any kind of history, you'll know that there has been a conspiracy to disharmonized the African people by all means. In this, they say that the Israelites are the chosen people.

However, during several invasions by the Roman Empire, Arabs and Greeks they ostracized the people of Canaan. Its seven nations had been conquered by the heathenistic heathens. Whereas; they claim to be scholars of the all knowing creator. The people of Canaan - Palestine migrated to Ithiopia and are known as the Falasha and Maasai Tribes. 1 Chronicles 9:12. Therefore; do not throw away your Bibles. Use them as a resource of learning it's mesleadings and misunderstandings regarding all people.

The Kaballah was devised after the Paut Neteru of Ancient Khamit, Canaan and Palestine! It was devised by the Endo-European and Arabizer.

Parapsychology and foreknowledge are two conceptions that differ within the realms of spirituality, setienism as well as hypocrisy. First of all, Affluenza as it relates to white supremacy, the wealthy and privileged individuals has continued to be a carcinogen towards racial classes of the minority as well as those who are at the lower class. This is where individuals tend to assume no responsibility for their negative behaviors and or actions.

They tend to pray for forgiveness after committing vile acts of lewdness, GLBT, crime and other forms of perversions. They have no understanding that they have never been given grace as the Bible mentions. The Bible wasn't written for all people. It was forbidden by slaves, immigrants and The African American. Also within the Constitution of The United States of America. You see religion has nothing at all to do with God. However; it has been used to manipulate and control the underprivileged and poor. You see, everyone has to suffer the consequences for their actions. However; all does not recognize and or understand the purpose for being.

The destiny is to be attained, comprehended and fulfilled. However; the Church and Mosque says pray or do a deed - / then you'll be forgiven for your sinful behavior-(s). However, this is a fallacy. Whereas; information does not heal the behavior / conditions of the affluenza type. You are only fooling yourselves if you believe tha Jesus Christ or Muhammad / Allah will save you.

The entire world is filled with the Affluenza Type individuals. They are easily swayed and are scapegoatable scapegoats who are willing and seeking whomever they can devour. Or whomever will devour them. These are psychiatric and paganistic fetishes. However; they aren't listed within the DSM. This leads individuals to assume that they'll never be convicted with GLBT, bullying, truancy, abortion, prostitution, psychiatrical conditioning, incest, rape, murder, theft, embezzlement, treason, expulsion, fraud and other malacious acts that are in violation of the universal and spiritual laws of the Paut Neteru.

There's no respector of persons with God! Therefore; beware of personal favortism. So, I must ask the following question. "Who is your personal saviour. You cannot have one. You see, God is a monotheistic God with a variety of spiritual and mental characteristics. This is where you govern yourselves by monitoring your own infirmities and psychiatrical - / behavioral conditions. Everyone is in the image of God. However; the majority are Affluenza type.

So you think that a civilization (Canaan - Khamit) of dignity can be ostracized for thousands of years without its slavers receiving spiritual consequences for the actions of their ancestors. That is Affluenza. Deuteronomy 28:29 of your King James Version of The Bible is for those type of individuals who are unwilling to cooperate with the universal laws of God!

Therefore; you cannot have it both ways. What I am saying is, individuals cannot worship the pagan religions of the Western civilization along with its pagan holidays, fornication and GLBT movements and also claim that they are non-racists and hypocratical towards race relations and aren't bigots. They are in denial, histrionic and narcisstic inwordly. They are ravaging wolves who resemble you and claim to be of you likeness.

You see, Afrocentricity is a lifestyle of the African and Afro-American. It isn't celebrated. It is lived. However; there are house-niggas who celebrate the paganistic ways - holidays- of the Western-man by attempting to live with, reside with and assemble with them. Their behaviors are then triggered upon others with patterns of molestation, rape, suicide, hatred, malice and murder. The majority of the people of the world are Type I and II Affluenza. You aren't saved or forgiven by a saviour. Therefore; you have been bewitched and bamboozled by the ministry and philosophies of the Setien.

In spirituality and psychiatry there are various forms of behaviour modification that must be ordained, comprehended, established, pursued and attained. In doing so, there is a form of self-discipline and self-actualization that is achieved. This goes beyond the Western civilized form of The Hierarchy of Needs and Multiple Intelligence of Garner and Maslow.

The Khamitic - Canaanite Tree of Life Meditation System shows no sign of Affluenza. You cannot be GLBT and claim their history within your private lives by living that particular lifestyle. That is the lower level of the sahu division. This is their lifestyle of vain imaginations. Whereas; 2Peter 1:20 No private intrepretation - no personal intrepretation and hidden agenda is the purpose of Gods' will within your life shall occur. It must be holisticly approached.

They seduce you with familiar spirits of WICCA, Christianity, Islam and Gay Tarot according to the Torah. Even though the Torah of Judiasm exposes Christianity, it has possessed Khamit and Canaan by treacherous forms of scheme. Therefore; how can individuals mention words, write books and preach sermons regarding race and racism if they haven't experienced as I have or as any other Afrocentric scholar has? Yet; they plagiarise the works of others by speaking parables that have been stolen from the Metu Neter, John Henrik Clarke and Dr. Ben Jochanan in order to sooth and please their congergations.

They have the Mary Leftkowitz Syndrome as well as being addicted to dark forms of hearsays by the Setien. For, they are scoffers! They claim Christ - Allah; yet they know that they're getting their knowledge from African Scholars and writers -; However; they marry into racists clans and families of European culture. Has not your bible told you about intermarriage. Read for yourselves. The Entire Old Testament does. There's no integration. There will always be seperation, hatred and discrimination. For, it is written! You have Affluenza!

Every living organism has to face consequence for received actions and interactions of all sorts. You are only fooling yourselves. Whereas; Job 1 mentions that Satan (Setien) was in the presence of the Lord. Humans of the world are affluenza type by the means of the flesh and imitating behaviors of others. For; they seek whomever they are capable of devouring. The Church and mosque are of setienistic that claim that they are in the presence of the Lord. You see; presence of the Lord could be any form of spiritual awaking. Such as; prayer, meditation, dreaming - realm sleep and or exorcism. Therefore; individuals have been observed in molesting the spirit and soul of another / others (the weak) with cunning forms of vile uses of idolatry. They seduce weak individuals with methodologies of cunning and clever designs of the Setien. For; they are aware of ones strengths and weaknesses. They are scavengers of the underworld and are in damnation. Will you join them.

Therefore; the Setien is anyone. Also, a member of a political party and clergy who is envious of others successes, anyone who is idle, lazy and a syllogical being. For this type of individual is willing to see the strong become weak by his or her constant negativities towards itself as well as others. In addition; The Naturalization Act of March 26th (Pagan holidays of Easter-Passover)1790 {the final day of Lent} was and is still currently geared to protect the Caucasian who were immigrants and were of good standing by forbidding The African, Indian and Asian Human and Civil Rights in The United States of America. 2 Thessalonoians 3:11 *1 Timothy 5:13 For they are busybodies and GLBT's.

Whereas: Thesalonica is located in Greece and so is Lesbos Island. Do you get my point. This episode is not out of Greece. For they were and are a people of carnality, hatred, cannabilism and greed. You see, it the so-called role of the sociologist to keep the community out of harms way. In this; many of them, like psychologist turn to carnal addictions, alcoholism, adultry, idolatry and depressions. This is due to them being trained and living the lifestyle and mindset of the of the slaver. That is, the Greek, Islamic, Christian and Indo-European way. Their ways has deterioated the Black community and entire African culture.

Mental Illness and race relations are entangled with theology, psychology and sociology as tactics of the setien as forms of dictation towards the lowly. In social behavior millions of individuals lack the positive abilities of social interaction due to the spiritual, sociological and psychological methods of western research. In this, there is racism, segregation, discrimination and hatred. Therefore; it is highly esteemed that the immigrant of the Naturalization Acts has often been the overly privileged. In the racist Book of James Chapter 2 of the King James Version of The Bible it mentions exactly what I am writing about.

Therefore; you cannot have it both ways. If you practice a certian religion, you cannot absorb (institute) others in order of soothing your flesh. You are then a hypocrate as well as a bigot as it relates to your own racist culture and cultural attitude towards The African and its decendents. Members of the clergy is well awasre of this. Yet, it is a whoremongering and environment of greed! It therefore; robs the blind with its use of words and cunning tactics of spiritual betrayal.

Many people of the African decent are too guilty by perjuring themselves is it relates to poor diet, abuses of drugs, alcohol, finances and sex as well as their unwillingness to utilize the Tree of Life Meditation properly. Many people of all races are lazy. They are willing to take short cuts. You too cannot have it both ways. You criticize; yet on the otherhand are afraid to awaken the shadows of your own dark behaviors that are within you by using human-shields / intercesseries to protect you. Setiens and heathens join aires. Therefore; conditions must be tamed spiritually.

Some individuals tend to be etreme by moving their furniture in spiritual directions during certain Khamitic cycles in order to dream and perform wickedness against the African during the cycle. This is their way by force - through rem sleep periods of continuing their lifestyle of the GLBT, fraud and demonology. You are only fooling yourselves. They are soldiers for the GLBT, adulterous and fonication lifestyles. For you judgement long time lingereth. 2 Peter 2:3. That's what your bible says.

For; it is written 2 Corinthians 5:20 that individuals are ambassaders of Christ must be reconciled with God. In Romans 1:30 It is written that many are haters of God. Therefore; you cannot have it both ways. You cannot be an ambassader of Christ and love God by committing malicious acts that will eliminate your person from the face of the universe. For the GLBT and the purpose sinner, there is no reconciliation. God and Christ aren't the same being. Christ is an image of the European slaver and God is the Almighty with a variety of characteristics and spiritual manifestations.

Man has fallen into darkness by abusing its ordained characteristics and manifestations. Therefore; those who are doomed and aren't redeemed. Leviticus 27:29. This is what Judiasm says. Is this the same Lord that is written in the same Bible regarding, the harlort, male prostitute, GLBT and or those who continue to commit spiritual and psychiatrical suicide. For they conspire to make you one of them. However; when it comes to suffering, /

you suffer alone. Alone without your peers in so-called Christianity. Surah 17:75 says this as for the Muslim too! You will be doomed during your entire life, death and after death. You'll have no ancestry for the destruction that you've created for yourself.

You cannot be reconcilled with God and be an ambassader for Christ. God is not a Christian or Muslim. You cannot have it both ways. You have been bewitched. You are fooling yourselves. Beware of personal favortism! Therefore; fornication is to have sexual intercourse prior to being married. Let's say this, what about the GLBT's. Aren't they too committing the same scheme? The same violation against the ordinances of God? They are of the gay community which is against the nature of God. The my girlfriend / my boyfriend and or my partner syndrome is an epidemic. They are too fornicating which is another violation against the psychiatrical and unconditioned nature of God.

They are without excuse. God is not a machine or beast that you can pound on with a hammer until he gives in like Kunta Kinte or others. Romans 1 as well as 1 Corinthians 6:9 says as well. You cannot have it both ways. Who is your saviour? Who is your prophet? Who is your messiah? Don't be inconsistent in your belief system. Also, you must understand that parapsychology and foreknowledge are similar in many instances. The two can harm you if you have no understanding of your true self and oneness with the creator within.

Whereas; their intent is to use your spiritual manifestations of the Tree of Life against you by invoking deities / deity (of your studies) towards your being in order to gain a greater divinity / knowledge for themselves. Therefore; their intent is to worship what they actually despise privily within their being of the House-Nigga / Caucasoid Setein. For they are angry within their persons and do not know or understand themselves. See Deuteronomy Chapter 28. In addition; they are fooling themselves. Their ways of seeking council are of conspiring against the lowly and humble through manipulating their higher qualities and convincing them that they are weak. This is the way of the racist, wicked and GLBT.

See Surah 17:75-77 which also has flaws. They too are guilty and false by committing malicious acts of genocide against ancient Khamit, Canaan and Palestine. Therefore; seek counsel from a griot, the true individual and storyteller of God!

HIDDEN HISTORICAL REFERENCES AND PREFERENCES

Racism, paganism and GLBT verses the historical facts and consciousness of the Ancient people of Africa, Cam / Khamit and the Bantu of the entire Sudan. Whereas; information will not heal you. From economics, moral issues, social issues, spirituality, healthcare and western medicine, man has been flawed into forms of mysterious fallacies with regards to his actual psychiatrical and medical condition(s). THUT The Thyroid Hormone Uptake Test has been a carcinogen towards the Black community as medical tests and exams have been created by names of ancient Egyptian pharoahs in order to continue to keep the so-called uneducated impoverished intellectually. Therefore; if you have no knowledge of your cultural history, you'll be defeated the the system of the Setien.

Animal toxicology is a form of racism that The WHO and its physicians have used for centuries to recondition, reshape and redefine their affluenza type of behaviour towards the African people. Whereas; the European, Christian, Greek, Jew and Arab has used religion and medicine to dictate and devalue the African and other minorities who have meager abilities to communicate by reading, speaking, writing and or making important decisions independantly. You see; The Naturalization Acts were not provided for the benefit of all races, cultures and nationalities. Seek counsel!

In fact, they were provided to extend all racial forms of ostracism. Ostracism is the banishment of citizens or a particular citizen by popular vote. Of course; this evolved in ancient Greece. The ancient Greeks and Romans Devised the Holy Bible. The Holy Bible is the number one selling book in the world. It is read with ignorance by the ignorant. There are no fact within it. The events within it has no factual evidents. It is quite syllogical. Therefore; what is said by deciding and judging what is true spiritually verses fallacies of biblical and religion based on what they have been told verses knowing through spiritual intervention and guidance by the universal laws has been misunderstood as a result of opionated busybodies who have not studied anything other than the Quran or King James Version of the Bible. This also includes Catholicism and the Catechist.

Indeed; those particular and popular religions had introduced us to all forms of slavery due to their arrogance in the forms of brainwashing, Arabizing and Christianizing our Civilization with a variety of dehumanizing tactics. As we invited them into our land they observed our ways,(mannerisms-conditions and behaviours) religions, spirituality, dietary habits, creations and lifestyles and conquered us - / then enslaved us with beheadings and maimings. They stole the wealth of our civilization by eroding our legacies and divinity with the twisting therof.

Individuals are filled with episodes of lies, logic and delusion when it comes to the understanding of spirtualality and themselves God! Individuals have itching ears and dangerous lips when it comes to their own heritage. This is to say that we must awaken our true selves by ignoring the outermost passions of churchianity and mosquanity by researching for ourselves and not by scoffing through hearsays of the wars of modernity and hatreds of the western and so-called middle eastern nations of seteinistic carcinogens of deceitfulness.

You see, Africa is the eldest of civilizations. Therefore; it is the melting pot and cradle of the universe. Karmah - Kerma of the northern Sudan was an ancient Egyptian colony in Kush, the modern of the Sudan. This includes the galaxies, celestials and other mysterious inhabitants. Everything was created by God and formed from within African culture. This includes spirituality and the true form of metaphysics that are occultable. However; whenever the word occult is used it is depicted the to undermind and shame the Black Man, Woman and Child. In addition; the education system doesn't make aware to its pupils of its authenticities of wealth and wholesomeness. Whereas; it has provided a consciousness that has shaken the the entire state of the European and Arab.

Dr. Hendric Clarke, Dr. Yosef A.A Ben-Jochannan and Ra Un Nefer Amen I has already exposed the philosphical and humiliating filth of the egotististic European and

Arab ministry. Whereas; primitive psychologists such as C. G. Jung and Richard Wilhelm researched the Bugishi districts of Uganda, Kenya and the Sudan in order to captivate and reconstruct what is known as the "Peculiar Institution" of the free and enslaved Negroe! This such activity continues to exist today. Whereas; individuals are currently institutionalized by the clergy, Iman and WHO for monetary and investigative research purposes.

In this; there is the hope that individuals will lose their cultural identity and knowledge of self in exchange for the pleasures of the mercenary. Indeed; Deuteronomy 28:25 The Lord will cause you to be defeated before you enemies. You will come at them from one direction but flee from them in seven. {This particular portion of the Bible denounces The Seven Nations of Canaan - The Promise Land} Whereas; it says "You will become a thing of horror to all of the kingdoms of the earth". You see; the Kaballah, which was derived from Canaan / Khamit was used in the Book of Deuteronomy. The 5 Books are of Judaism. Whereas; The Book of Genesis was written after the fact.

Deuteronomy 18:10 deals with REPITITION COMPULSION DISORDER as it relates to individuals observing times repiticiously and negatively. Their initial intent is to invoke other individuals to carry out their activities through intercessary, on behalf of others. In addition; verses 10 through 12 also deals with racial issues that the European, Jew, Greek and Arab that has been conjured in order to save their own souls throughout Islam, Judaism and Christianity. This is where the denial of African Ancestry is initiated in order to maintain the dictatorship of those who are of the lack of understanding regarding spirituality, racial issues and themselves. Therefore; if you use the Bible or Quran as your religious outlook and live by their standards, you are living in hipocrisy and are a Setien. If it is written - you must abide according to your doctrine of belief.

7 directions: Deuteronomy 28:25 {repitition compulsion} is also known as{Autism Spectrum Disorder} in the DSM. This can be a self-inflicted disorder as well the Schizotypal Personality Disorder. The two are coined as slightly similar to the point where individuals feel that they have magical powers over others through manipulation and scheme. You see, the western civilization as well as its religious affiliates has often penalized the meek by representing the holier then now spectrum of individuals. In this, oracles were used several

time throughout the Old Testament by priest of Judaism. However; the use has been sanctioned by the European who had conquered the Seven Nations of Canaan.

The European and Arabic cultures have used tarot astrology in order to read the fate of a nation with regards to the non-development of spiritual awareness. However; The Oracle of Baal was used throughout Canaan, Egypt, the Sudan and the majority of Africa to fertilize the dynasties, cultures and inhabitants. In addition, it is said that Canaan will scatter in seven directions. The seven nations of The Promise Land of Canaan were the following prior to post colonialism periods by the people of Shem and Japheth;

1. Canaanites -Kenaanim
2. Hittites - Chittim
3. Hivites - Chivvim
4. Perrizites - Perizzim
5. Girgashites - Girgasim
6. Amorites - Emorim
7. Jebusites - Yebusim

Which is deliberate racism and ostracism. Whereas; the nations of Canaan were considered detestable pagans as a result of being spiritually gifted with a great deal of creation, wisdom and intellect. Whereas; this is a theory of scapegoating by the Egyptologist, mercenary, psychologist and so-called irrational biblical scholar who has been deceitful as to opposing the greatness of ancient Egypt, Palestine and Canaan. This includes the greatness of any person of color.

The point that I am trying to make is as follows; The Khamitic Tree of Life System is based on the aspects too of ancient Canaan. This of which was not used for the purposes of astrological, fortunetelling and zodialogical preferences for the purpose of horoscope reading. However; on the otherhand, Schizotypal Personality Disorder and Repititious Compulsion Disorder have been determined By Sigmund Freud and The American Psychiatric Association based on racist methods of technological research of questionable procedural forms of animal and inhumane techniques of toxicology.

Therefore; African spirituality is to enhance ones totality. Ones entire spiritual and mental well-being. However; the Egyptologist, European, Jew, Christian and Arab has used colonistic slurs against it. This has lead to a depression within african villages as previously written with regards to the I-Ching, Jung and Wilheilm. In addition; animism was a part of the lives of the Sudanese and man of Egyptian Nubia. This also includes the mid and southern sections of Africa.

Whereas; Genesis 1:27 Man is considered in the image of God. However; Ecclesiastes 7:29 says "God created mankind upright, but they have gone in search of many schemes" through dissuasion. This is where rasicms and greed has manifested by the slaver and manipulator of the lowly and or lower spirited individuals. In this; dissuasion is not a mystery towards the ancient as well as modern tribesmen. Whereas; leaders have been dissuaded into giving up their vision and universal purpose through a variety of forms of lies, bribery and conspiracy. For example; there are Chronicles 9:12 was a tribe of war during the reign of King David.

However; The Maasai Tribe is of Kenya, Ethiopia and the Sudan. Indeed; it has been written that the Falasha Jews migrated from Israel to Ethiopia and to the Promise Land during the invasions by the Egyptians during the time of Moses. The Promise Land was the Seven Nations of Canaan. During this modern day, those particular nations are under Christian, Jewish and Islamic rule as a result of colonistic methods of manipulation and dissuasion.

This has become a ritualistic form of spiritual and psychiatrical conditioning that has that has been caused by tha allegorical themes of religion. Whereas; this has been written within the Holy Bible as well as the Holy Quran. In Galatians 4:24 it mentions allegorical as it pertains to a women being in bondage as well as being liberated into freedom. That is the Jew, arab and modern (Egyptian). They have no clue. Surah 3:7 He it is who revealed the Book to thee: some of the verses are decisive -- they are on the basis of the book --- others are allegorical. Then those in whose hearts are of perversity follow the part of it which is allegorical. They are and have been seeking to mislead. and seeking to give it (their own) interpretation.

Note: the fact that an allegorical is a story that has a deeper or more general meaning. Which is a figure of speech and a form of general ideas. All of which leads to various forms of psychological ideation. A fabrication of ideas. Whereas; words tend to become twisted. Deuteronomy 16:19 do not pervert justice or show partiality. Do not accept a bribe. For a bribe blinds the eyes of the wise and twists the words of the innocent. A bribe is to persuade one to act in ones favor or commit illegal acts of behaviour. You'll then become a By-Word, which is a person or thing which is cited for a notorious and outstanding example of the embodiment of something as a result of his or her idolatrous principals. Deuteronomy 28:37 you will become a thing of horror, a by word and an object of ridicule among the peoples where the Lord will drive you.

CHILDREN OF A CURSE

I n Demonic Pathology ----- Acts 17:11 with regards to the law of generations {generational curses} as forementioned in Deuteronomy 28:18 says 'Cursed is the fruit of your womb'. Therefore; there is no psychiatrical cure for those who are cursed and are doomed. For none that are devoted unto men, but they are doomed and are not to be redeemed. Parents have begotten children who are set to be doomed as well through, pedophillia, child inticement, abortion, incest, child endangerment, gender disorders, sexisms and racisms.

For they are children of a curse as written in 2 Peter 2:14. In this; which is non-contrawise towards the words of Jesus {Serapis}. Whereas; this has led to the above forementioned message. Matthew 19:14-15 Jesus said to the children "Come Unto Me"! Hinder them not! You see, Jesus has been depicted as a White Man for thousands of years through deception. Have you forgotten, Christianity, judaism and Islam has been greatly markeded as the "cream of the crop" religions. In this Come Unto Me is a representation of the so-called fall of Sodom and Gomorrah.

Whereas; {to come unto} is to ejaculate upon another! You get my point about pedophillia and the GLBT movenents. You see, The Bible is allegorical filled with fallacies, delusions and filthy lies of plagarisms and deceit. 1 Timothy 5:22 (do not hasty lay hands on anyone) Huh! Suffer no more equates to effiminisms and idolatries of foreign forces and powers of monarchy as well as dictatorship. Isaiah 30:1 "Woe" to the obstinate - Children - Nation - those who carry out plans that aren't mine. Forming an alliance, but not by my spirit, heaping sin upon sin.

This reveals the deceptions against the nations of Canaan. It says in Isaiah 1:2 I reared up children {nations} and brought them up, but they have rebelled against me. Therefore; through obstinate and rebellious children, that is how religions and occultic activities are developed by pastors, clerics and priests. The lowly is seduced through brainwashing. Individuals become members of Isis, Al Qaeda, Boko Haram and Al Shebab. You see, children become gang members, GLBT's as well as murderous and suicidal.

You are Children of a Curse carries a lot of weight. this is through inconsistent forms and methods of behavioral modifications. whereas; information will not cure negative mental and spitirual conditions and so - on. Educators are distracted as they seek monetary gain and reward for their teaching abilities. They are sheep in wolves clothings. As they are detractractors, distractors, destractive and unstable in their own philosophical forms of rational thinking.

Note: It is through peer pressures and unique schemes of bullying that children become involved in inappropriate relationships that includes destructive behaviors through intercessary prayer by their parents and the so-called educated fool. Intercession will not save the culprits who are conditioned with negative externalized behaviors and modifications which are racially biased through religious bigotry and favortisms.

The pathology of negative behavior is psychopathology. Psychopathology is a the study of mental disorders. this includes efforts to understand their biological, psychological, social, economical, physiological and genetic causes.

Psyche = soul / Pathos = suffering as ology = wholly. This is taken from the Euro-Greek form of philosophy and psychology. This is racism in a nutshell. Conditioned and uncontrol-able behavioral patterns tend to trigger as does STD's. Deuteronomy 28:61 You will have diseases that are and will be uncurable. In addition; many mental illnesses are due to other medical conditions - {ICD} This includes substance induced disorders such as: Organic hallucinations as well as organic delusional disorders which relates to Tourettes Syndrome and Autism. The two are related due to generational curses due the drug abuses, anxieties and repitition compulsions.

Note: generational curses equates to Surah (17:75-77). This is of which they have ignored the positive attributes by the notable people of Ancient Kemet and Canaan! In this; there's are factors of drug abuse - sexual addictions, cultural imitations - of racial tendencies and spiritual idolatry. This is also where they formed the 7 Churches of Asia - THE GREEKS -: and dehumanized the 7 Nations of Canaan. Whereas; third world countries have suffered {Africa} and have been induced with ill-curable diseases and disorders of the STD, psychiatric and genetic carcinogens that are pathological and demoralizing to a certain culture and nation of people.

This has led to a history of mythology. In mythology, there has been allegorical schemes to exclude the legacy of the people of ancient Kemet, ways in which racism has evolved and the psychiatrical, physiological and biological factors of the GLBT movements.

* 9 7 8 1 4 9 0 7 7 0 3 4 5 *